I0116617

NOBODY TOLD ME

HIDDEN TRUTHS ABOUT UNHEALTHY FOODS IN AMERICA AND THEIR LINK TO DISEASES

MOHAMED IDDRISU

Nobody Told Me

Copyright © 2025 by Mohamed Iddrisu.

All rights reserved. No part of this publication may be reproduced, distributed, or transmitted in any form or by any means, including photocopying, recording, or other electronic or mechanical methods, without the written consent of the publisher. The only exceptions are for brief quotations included in critical reviews and other noncommercial uses permitted by copyright law.

MILTON & HUGO L.L.C.
4407 Park Ave., Suite 5
Union City, NJ 07087, USA

Website: *www. miltonandhugo.com*
Hotline: *1- 888-778-0033*
Email: *info@miltonandhugo.com*

Ordering Information:
Quantity sales. Special discounts are granted to corporations, associations, and other organizations. For more information on these discounts, please reach out to the publisher using the contact information provided above.

Library of Congress Control Number: 2025912138
ISBN-13:   979-8-89285-473-3   [Paperback Edition]
                    979-8-89285-472-6   [Digital Edition]

Rev. date: 06/09/2025

For everyone who deserve to know the truth about their food.
And for the dreamers who believe change is possible.

CONTENTS

ACKNOWLEDGMENTS

This book is the culmination of years of research, conversations, and personal reflection. I owe my deepest gratitude to those who inspired and supported me throughout this process.

To my family: Your encouragement and belief in me fueled this journey.

To the researchers, activists, and health professionals who are challenging the status quo of the food industry: Thank you for your courage and dedication.

To my readers: This book is for you. Thank you for being willing to open your minds and take control of your health.

PREFACE

"Why didn't anyone tell me?"

These words echoed in my mind the day I discovered the truth about the food I had trusted for years. Like many, I believed that labels like "low-fat" or "natural" meant healthy, that fast food was an occasional indulgence with no long-term consequences, and that the American food system was designed to nourish us. I was wrong.

This book is not just about my journey—it's about the journey we are all on as consumers navigating a minefield of misinformation. It's about empowering ourselves to question, learn, and act. Together, we will uncover hidden truths, confront uncomfortable realities, and take the first steps toward a healthier, more informed future.

CHAPTER

1

The Food Illusion

Food in America isn't what it seems. Every aisle of the supermarket is a carefully curated illusion, a stage where products are dressed in costumes of trust and health to play their part in the grand theater of consumer deception. Buzzwords like "organic," "gluten-free," and "all-natural" dominate the packaging, whispering assurances to harried shoppers that what they're buying is not just good for their bodies but also aligned with their values. But peel back the layers, and you'll find a web of half-truths, outright lies, and an industry that thrives on manipulation.

The Hidden Agenda of the Supermarket

When you walk into a supermarket, you're entering a meticulously designed environment. Every shelf, every label, every product placement is engineered to guide your choices. Eye-level shelves? Reserved for the most profitable items, often not the healthiest ones. End caps (the displays at the ends of aisles)? Frequently showcase products high in sugar, salt, and fat because these are the items that sell—and bring the most revenue.

Take the cereal aisle, for example. Boxes shout out claims like "whole grain" or "high in fiber," giving the impression of health and nutrition.

But flip that box over and read the ingredients list. What you're likely to find is a cocktail of refined sugars, artificial flavors, and minimal whole grains. Some cereals marketed to children, with their colorful mascots and cartoon characters, contain more sugar per serving than a candy bar. Yet, parents buy these products, reassured by the health claims plastered across the front of the box.

It's not just cereal. Consider the so-called "healthy" frozen meals. They promise convenience without compromise, boasting low calories or fat-free ingredients. But delve into the fine print, and you'll discover meals packed with sodium—sometimes upwards of 1,000 milligrams per serving—to compensate for flavor lost in the processing. Additives like preservatives and artificial flavorings help extend shelf life, but what do they do to your body over time?

The Language of Deception

The food industry has mastered the art of linguistic manipulation. Words like "natural" carry no formal FDA (Food and Drug Administration) definition, yet they evoke a sense of wholesomeness. A bag of chips labeled "natural" is still fried in oils that contribute to heart disease. The term "organic" can be used loosely in processed foods that, while meeting certain standards, are still loaded with sugar and fat. "Gluten-free"? It sounds healthy but has no bearing on nutritional value for people who don't have celiac disease or gluten sensitivities. Even the colors on the packaging play a psychological role. Green suggests health, vitality, and nature. A loaf of bread in green packaging might sell better than the same loaf in a white wrapper simply because of the subconscious association with freshness and health.

The Psychology of the Illusion

The deception doesn't stop at words and images—it's rooted in psychology. Most consumers don't have the time, energy, or expertise to scrutinize every label. The food industry knows this. It exploits our fast-paced lives, offering convenience as the ultimate selling point. The promise of a quick meal that's "good for you" is irresistible to someone juggling work, family, and countless other responsibilities.

Moreover, the industry preys on emotions. Nostalgia is a powerful marketing tool. That "classic" macaroni-and-cheese brand may remind you of childhood dinners even though it's now loaded with more artificial ingredients than it had decades ago. Similarly, ads for "family-sized" snacks evoke images of togetherness, cleverly masking the fact that these oversized portions contribute to overeating.

The Cost of Convenience

For decades, Americans have prioritized convenience over quality. Fast food, microwave dinners, and packaged snacks dominate our diets. Yet this convenience comes at a cost—in terms of both money and health. Obesity rates have soared, as have cases of diabetes, heart disease, and other diet-related illnesses. The irony is that many of these "convenient" foods are priced higher than their less-processed counterparts. A bag of precut fruit costs significantly more than a whole fruit, even though the labor saved is minimal. Similarly, a box of sugary cereal often costs more per ounce than a bag of oats. The illusion of convenience masks the fact that we're paying a premium for unhealthy options.

Behind the Curtain: Big Food and Big Money

At the heart of the food illusion is an industry driven by profit. Major corporations spend billions on advertising designed to influence our choices. They fund studies that cast their products in a favorable light, often skewing the data to downplay health risks. They lobby policymakers to avoid regulations that could threaten their bottom line. Take the case of sugar. Decades ago, the sugar industry funded research that shifted the blame for heart disease onto fats, diverting attention from the role of sugar. The result? Generations of Americans were told to avoid butter and eggs while consuming low-fat products loaded with added sugars. This misinformation has had devastating consequences for public health.

The power of the food industry extends beyond advertising and research. It also shapes our dietary guidelines. Many of the organizations responsible for these guidelines receive funding from food corporations, creating conflicts of interest. Is it any wonder that the recommendations often align with industry interests rather than public health?

The Emotional Toll

The food illusion isn't just a public health issue—it's also a deeply personal one. Many Americans feel guilt and shame about their eating habits, believing they are failing to make healthy choices. But the reality is that the system is rigged against them. From childhood, we're conditioned to crave sugary, salty, and fatty foods. We're bombarded with advertisements that blur the line between indulgence and necessity.

Parents, in particular, face an emotional burden. They want to feed their children healthy meals but are often misled by marketing claims. The guilt of unknowingly serving processed foods disguised as healthy options weighs heavily, creating a cycle of frustration and helplessness.

Breaking Free from the Illusion

Awareness is the first step toward breaking free from the food illusion. By understanding how the system works, we can make more informed choices. This doesn't mean overhauling your entire diet overnight—it's about small, conscious changes. Read labels carefully. Look beyond the buzzwords and examine the ingredients list. Prioritize whole, unprocessed foods when possible.

Education is another crucial component. The more we learn about nutrition, the harder it becomes for the industry to deceive us. Sharing this knowledge with others can create a ripple effect, empowering communities to demand transparency and accountability.

A Glimmer of Hope

Despite the overwhelming influence of the food industry, there's a growing movement toward healthier, more sustainable eating habits. Farmers' markets, community-supported agriculture (CSA) programs, and local co-ops are becoming more accessible. Consumers are beginning to question the status quo, pushing for clearer labeling and more honest marketing practices.

The food illusion may be pervasive, but it's not unbreakable. By uncovering the truth and making intentional choices, we can reclaim control over our diets and our health. The journey begins not in the supermarket aisles but in our minds as we learn to see through the carefully constructed façade and recognize food for what it truly is.

The deception runs deep, but the path to empowerment is clear. In the chapters that follow, we will explore the origins of this illusion, the science behind our cravings, and the steps we can take to build a healthier, more authentic relationship with food. The question is, are you ready to uncover the truth?

CHAPTER

2

The Rise of Processed Foods

Processed foods have become a ubiquitous part of the American diet, offering convenience, affordability, and indulgence. Yet their rise has been far from inevitable. The story of how processed foods transformed the way we eat is one of industrial innovation, marketing genius, and unintended consequences. From the factories of post–World War II America to today's supermarkets lined with colorful packages, the evolution of processed foods reflects a broader cultural shift toward convenience and mass production—but at a profound cost.

A Postwar Revolution in Food

The origins of modern processed foods can be traced back to World War II. During the war, the United States invested heavily in technologies that create long-lasting, transportable food supplies for soldiers. Canned goods, powdered milk, and instant coffee were staples on the battlefield. These innovations were lifesaving during wartime, but when the war ended, manufacturers faced a new challenge: what to do with these technologies in peacetime.

Enter the burgeoning consumer economy of the 1950s. With soldiers returning home and women encouraged to leave the workforce to focus on domestic life, the stage was set for the rise of convenience foods.

Companies rebranded their wartime products as modern kitchen staples, promising to make life easier for the emerging middle class. Instant mashed potatoes, boxed cake mixes, and frozen TV dinners were marketed as miracles of modern science.

Behind the scenes, however, food scientists weren't just preserving food—they were engineering it. Techniques like hydrogenation, emulsification, and freeze-drying allowed manufacturers to create products with extended shelf lives and uniform textures. These processes also made food cheap to produce and easy to distribute.

But these innovations came at a cost. Natural ingredients were replaced with synthetic substitutes. Real sugar gave way to high-fructose corn syrup, and butter was swapped for margarine loaded with trans fats. While these changes made processed foods more affordable, they also introduced substances into the American diet that our bodies were never designed to handle.

The Truth about "Convenience"

The rise of processed foods didn't just reshape diets—it redefined what food meant to Americans. Convenience became a key selling point, and food manufacturers worked tirelessly to align their products with this value. Commercials portrayed smiling housewives serving up casseroles made with condensed soup, while colorful advertisements promised that new snacks would delight children and free up mothers' time.

But was it really about convenience, or was it about control? By engineering foods to last longer, taste more addictive, and cost less to produce, food corporations fundamentally shifted the balance of power in the food system. Farmers were relegated to producing raw ingredients for an industrial supply chain while consumers became increasingly disconnected from the origins of their food.

Even more troubling was the way these foods were designed. Processed foods are not just preserved—they are engineered to maximize profits. This means they are carefully formulated to hit what scientists call the *bliss point*—the perfect balance of sugar, salt, and fat that triggers pleasure responses in the brain. These foods don't just satisfy hunger—they create cravings, leading to overconsumption and addiction-like behavior.

Myths of Nutrition and Health

One of the great myths perpetuated by the processed-food industry is that its products are nutritionally equivalent—or even superior—to whole foods. Early marketing campaigns boasted of added vitamins and minerals, suggesting that processed foods were the modern solution to nutritional deficiencies. Breakfast cereals, for instance, were often touted as "fortified" with essential nutrients despite being loaded with sugar.

This myth has been thoroughly debunked by science. Whole foods, such as fresh fruits, vegetables, and grains, provide a complex array of nutrients that work synergistically to promote health. Processed foods, on the other hand, often strip these natural nutrients away during production, replacing them with synthetic additives that fail to replicate the benefits of real food.

Consider bread: Traditional bread, made from just a few simple ingredients, is a wholesome staple. But mass-produced bread is a different story. To extend shelf life and improve texture, manufacturers remove the wheat germ and bran during processing, stripping the bread of fiber and nutrients. Then they add back a handful of synthetic vitamins and call it "enriched." While the product might meet basic nutritional guidelines, it pales in comparison to the benefits of whole-grain bread.

The Hidden Costs of Processed Foods

The rise of processed foods has had devastating consequences for public health. Rates of obesity, diabetes, and heart disease have skyrocketed, driven in part by diets high in sugar, trans fats, and sodium—all hallmarks of processed foods. The correlation is hard to ignore: As processed food consumption has increased, so too have the incidences of these chronic diseases.

High-fructose corn syrup is one of the most infamous culprits. Introduced in the 1970s as a cheap alternative to sugar, it became a staple in everything from sodas to salad dressings. But studies have shown that high-fructose corn syrup is metabolized differently than regular sugar, leading to increased fat storage and a greater risk of metabolic disorders.

Then there are the artificial additives—preservatives, flavorings, and colorings—that give processed foods their signature look and taste. While many of these additives are approved by regulatory agencies, their long-term health effects are not fully understood. Some, like artificial food dyes, have been linked to hyperactivity in children, while others may contribute to inflammation and other health issues.

Emotional Connections and Cultural Shifts

The dominance of processed foods has not only altered our diets, it has also reshaped our relationship with food. For many Americans, these products are deeply nostalgic. A box of macaroni and cheese, a frozen pizza, or a can of soda evokes memories of childhood comfort and family gatherings. Food manufacturers have capitalized on this emotional connection, using marketing campaigns to position their products as symbols of love, happiness, and tradition.

Yet this nostalgia often masks a deeper loss. As processed foods became more prevalent, traditional cooking practices fell by the wayside. Families spent less time preparing meals together, and the art of cooking was increasingly outsourced to factories and corporations. The rise of convenience food coincided with a decline in culinary skills, leaving many people dependent on packaged meals.

Myths vs. Reality

The processed-food industry has perpetuated numerous myths to maintain its dominance. One persistent myth is that cooking from scratch is too time-consuming for modern families. Yet studies have shown that preparing a simple, healthy meal at home can take less time than ordering takeout or heating up a frozen dinner.

Another myth is that processed foods are more affordable than fresh, whole foods. While it's true that some processed foods are cheaper upfront, they often come with hidden costs. Poor nutrition leads to higher health-care expenses while overconsumption contributes to obesity and other chronic conditions. In the long run, these costs far outweigh the savings at the checkout counter.

Reclaiming Our Diets

Understanding the history of processed foods is the first step toward reclaiming our diets. By recognizing the forces that shaped the modern food landscape, we can begin to make more informed choices about what we eat. This doesn't mean rejecting all convenience foods—after all, some degree of processing is necessary to feed a growing population. But it does mean prioritizing whole, minimally processed foods whenever possible.

It also means questioning the narratives we've been sold. Convenience is not inherently bad, but it shouldn't come at the expense of our health or the environment. By learning to cook, growing our food, or supporting local farmers, we can take back control of our food systems and reconnect with the joy of eating real, nourishing food.

The rise of processed foods is a cautionary tale about the unintended consequences of industrial innovation. What began as a solution to wartime shortages has become a public health crisis, fueled by a culture of convenience and profit-driven corporations.

But it's not too late to turn the tide. By embracing the truths about food and rejecting the myths, we can pave the way for a healthier, more sustainable future.

CHAPTER

3

The Sugar Trap

Sugar is everywhere. It's not just in the obvious places—cookies, candies, and sodas—but also in the unexpected ones, like whole wheat bread, salad dressings, yogurt, and even "health" foods like granola bars and protein shakes. For decades, the food industry has wielded sugar as its secret weapon, exploiting its addictive properties to drive sales and consumer loyalty. Cheap, versatile, and highly palatable, sugar has become a cornerstone of the modern diet. But the cost of our collective sweet tooth is staggering.

Behind the glossy advertisements and irresistible flavors lies a darker truth: Sugar isn't just a harmless indulgence—it's a driver of addiction, a contributor to chronic disease, and a disruptor of our biological systems. By understanding the science, history, and marketing tactics behind sugar, we can begin to break free from its grip.

The Science of Sugar Addiction

When you eat sugar, your brain responds as if it's receiving a reward. The sweet taste activates dopamine release in the brain's reward system, triggering feelings of pleasure and satisfaction. This is the same mechanism triggered by drugs like cocaine and nicotine, albeit to a lesser degree. Over time, repeated consumption of sugar leads to desensitization—your brain releases less dopamine in response, requiring you to consume more to achieve the same effect.

This phenomenon, known as tolerance, is a hallmark of addiction. It's why you might start with a single cookie but find yourself unable to stop after eating half the box.

Studies have shown that sugar not only stimulates the brain's reward centers, it can also alter its wiring, turning cravings and overconsumption into a deeply ingrained habit.

The Biological Impact of Sugar

The effects of sugar addiction aren't confined to the brain. Excessive sugar wreaks havoc on the body in multiple ways:

1. Blood sugar spikes and crashes

When you consume sugar, it rapidly enters your bloodstream, causing a spike in your blood sugar levels. This triggers a surge of insulin, the hormone responsible for regulating blood sugar. The subsequent crash leaves you feeling tired, irritable, and craving more sugar—creating a vicious cycle.

2. Fat storage and weight gain

Excess sugar that isn't immediately used for energy is stored as fat, often around the liver and abdomen. High sugar consumption is a key driver of obesity, particularly due to the prevalence of sugary beverages that don't trigger feelings of fullness, leading to overconsumption.

3. Chronic diseases

Over time, a high-sugar diet can lead to insulin resistance, a precursor to type 2 diabetes. It also contributes to inflammation, a root cause of heart disease, cancer, and other chronic illnesses.

4. Liver damage

Fructose, a component of sugar, is metabolized by the liver. When consumed in excess, it overwhelms the liver, leading to fat accumulation and, in severe cases, non-alcoholic fatty liver disease (NAFLD).

The Hidden Sugars in Our Diets

One of the most insidious aspects of sugar is how it's hidden in foods we wouldn't expect. In the 1970s and 1980s, as dietary fat became public enemy number one, food manufacturers scrambled to create low-fat products that still tasted good. Their solution? Add sugar.

Today, sugar lurks in nearly three-quarters of packaged foods under a variety of disguises. It's listed on ingredient labels under names like sucrose, fructose, dextrose, maltose, and high-fructose corn syrup (HFCS). Less obvious culprits include ingredients like honey, agave nectar, and fruit juice concentrate, which, despite their "natural" labels, have similar effects on blood sugar and insulin.

Consider these examples:

Yogurt. A single serving of flavored yogurt can contain as much sugar as a candy bar.

Bread. Many loaves, even those labeled "whole grain," include added sugars to enhance flavor and texture.

Sauces and condiments. Ketchup, barbecue sauce, and salad dressings are often loaded with sugar to balance acidity or enhance taste.

The Daily Sugar Overload

The World Health Organization (WHO) recommends that added sugars comprise no more than 10 percent of daily caloric intake, with an ideal target of 5 percent—about 25 grams (6 teaspoons) for most adults. Yet the average American consumes nearly three times this amount.

Children are especially vulnerable. Sweetened cereals, fruit juices, and snack bars marketed as "healthy" often contain more sugar than parents realize. Early exposure to sugary foods can set the stage for lifelong preferences and addiction, making it even harder to break the cycle.

The Role of the Food Industry

The pervasiveness of sugar in the modern diet isn't accidental—it's the result of deliberate choices by the food industry. Sugar is cheap to produce, enhances flavor, and extends shelf life, making it a favorite ingredient for manufacturers.

Perhaps most alarming is the way companies exploit sugar's addictive qualities. Through intensive research, food scientists have perfected the bliss point—the exact combination of sugar, salt, and fat that makes a product irresistible. The goal isn't to satisfy hunger but to keep you coming back for more.

In the 1980s, internal documents from the sugar industry revealed a concerted effort to downplay the health risks of sugar while shifting the blame for obesity and heart disease onto dietary fat. This misinformation campaign influenced decades of dietary guidelines, misleading consumers and perpetuating the myth that low-fat, high-sugar foods were healthy.

Truths and Myths about Sugar

Myth 1: Sugar is just empty calories.

While it's true that sugar lacks essential nutrients, its effects go far beyond providing "empty calories." Excess sugar actively harms the body by contributing to metabolic dysfunction, inflammation, and hormonal imbalances.

Myth 2: Natural sugars are healthier.

Sugars found in honey, maple syrup, and coconut sugar may contain trace minerals, but their impact on blood sugar and insulin is nearly identical to that of refined sugar. Whole fruits, by contrast, are healthier because they contain fiber, which slows sugar absorption.

Myth 3: Artificial sweeteners are a safe alternative.

Artificial sweeteners like aspartame, sucralose, and saccharin are marketed as healthier substitutes, but their safety is controversial. Some studies suggest they may disrupt gut bacteria, increase cravings for sweet foods, and even contribute to weight gain.

The Emotional Toll of Sugar Addiction

For many people, sugar isn't just a dietary habit—it's an emotional crutch. From childhood birthday cakes to comfort foods during stressful times, sugar is deeply intertwined with our emotions and memories.

This emotional connection can make reducing sugar intake feel like a loss. It's not just about giving up a flavor—it's about confronting the role that sugar plays in our lives, from celebrations to coping mechanisms.

The food industry capitalizes on this emotional bond, using marketing to associate sugary products with happiness, love, and reward. Advertisements for sugary cereals show families bonding over breakfast, while candy commercials promise joy and indulgence. These messages reinforce our dependence on sugar, making it harder to let go.

Breaking Free from the Sugar Trap

Escaping the sugar trap requires a combination of awareness, planning, and perseverance. Here are some strategies:

1. Read labels carefully.

Look for hidden sugars in ingredient lists, and be aware of alternative names like glucose, maltodextrin, and cane syrup.

2. Prioritize whole foods.

Focus on eating whole, unprocessed foods like vegetables, fruits, whole grains, and lean proteins.

3. Limit sugary beverages.

Sodas, energy drinks, and even fruit juices are major sources of added sugar. Replace them with water, herbal tea, or unsweetened beverages.

4. Balance your meals.

Pairing carbohydrates with protein and healthy fats can help stabilize blood sugar levels and reduce cravings.

5. Practice mindful eating.

Pay attention to your hunger cues and emotional triggers. Eating slowly and savoring your food can help you break the cycle of mindless consumption.

6. Find alternatives.

Satisfy your sweet tooth with natural options like whole fruit, or try spices like cinnamon and vanilla to add flavor without sugar.

A Path Forward

The sugar trap is deeply embedded in modern culture, but change is possible. By educating ourselves about the dangers of sugar and making conscious choices about what we eat, we can reclaim our health and break free from its grip.

This journey is not just about avoiding sugar—it's about rediscovering the joy of real, nourishing food. It's about challenging the narratives that have kept us hooked and embracing a lifestyle that prioritizes well-being over convenience.

Sugar may be a powerful force, but our ability to take control of our diets is stronger. The path forward starts with a single choice—and that choice can lead to a lifetime of better health and freedom.

CHAPTER

4

Fat Facts and Fictions

For years, fat has been the scapegoat of dietary health crises, blamed for expanding waistlines, clogged arteries, and heart disease. By the mid-twentieth century, nutrition advice vilified fats, sparking a wave of low-fat and fat-free products to flood the market.

These products, touted as healthier alternatives, often replaced fats with sugar, refined carbohydrates, and artificial additives, ironically exacerbating the very health issues they claimed to solve.

Yet, as science has advanced, so has our understanding of fats. Not all fats are created equal, and some are not only beneficial but essential for our health. Healthy fats provide critical nutrients, fuel our bodies, and protect us against chronic disease. On the other hand, harmful fats, like trans fats and hydrogenated oils, contribute to a host of health problems.

This chapter dives deep into the facts and fictions surrounding fats. From unraveling their tarnished reputation to celebrating their vital role in our diets, it's time to set the record straight.

The Rise and Fall of Fat: A Historical Perspective

In the mid-twentieth century, a war on fat was declared, and its origins can be traced to a mix of flawed science and public health panic.

The tipping point came in the 1950s when physiologist Ancel Keys introduced his Seven Countries Study, linking dietary fat—particularly saturated fat—to heart disease. Keys's work was influential, but his conclusions were based on selective data, ignoring countries where high-fat diets didn't correlate with high rates of heart disease.

The research gained momentum, culminating in the 1977 Dietary Goals for the United States, which recommended reducing fat intake and prioritizing carbohydrates. Food manufacturers capitalized on this directive, creating low-fat and fat-free versions of everything from yogurt to cookies. But removing fat meant sacrificing flavor, so sugar and artificial fillers were added to compensate.

The result? A paradoxical health crisis. While fat consumption dropped, obesity and diabetes rates soared. The low-fat craze demonized all fats, leaving consumers confused and unknowingly consuming excessive amounts of sugar and processed carbohydrates—factors now recognized as major contributors to chronic disease.

The Truth about Fats

Fats are not inherently harmful. In fact, they are a critical macronutrient that plays a vital role in our bodies. They provide energy, support cell structure, assist in nutrient absorption, and help produce essential hormones. The key is understanding the different types of fats and their effects on health.

The Good Fats

1. Monounsaturated fats

Found in: Olive oil, avocados, nuts, and seeds

Benefits: Monounsaturated fats are heart-healthy, helping to reduce LDL (low-density lipoprotein), or "bad" cholesterol, while maintaining HDL (high-density lipoprotein), or "good" cholesterol. They also improve insulin sensitivity, reducing the risk of type 2 diabetes.

2. Polyunsaturated fats

Found in: Fatty fish (like salmon, mackerel, and sardines), walnuts, flaxseeds, and sunflower oil

Benefits: These fats include omega-3 and omega-6 fatty acids, essential nutrients the body cannot produce on its own. Omega-3s, in particular, are anti-inflammatory and support brain health, heart health, and joint function.

The Bad Fats

1. Saturated fats

Found in: Butter, cheese, red meat, and coconut oil

Debate: Saturated fats have long been blamed for raising cholesterol levels and increasing heart disease risk. However, recent research suggests the relationship is more complex. While excessive saturated fat intake can be harmful, moderate consumption, particularly from whole, minimally processed foods, may not be as detrimental as once thought.

2. Trans fats

Found in: Margarine, shortening, and processed baked goods (like cookies, cakes, and crackers)

Danger: Trans fats are created through hydrogenation, a process that turns liquid oils into solid fats to extend shelf life. These fats are unequivocally harmful, raising LDL cholesterol, lowering HDL cholesterol, and significantly increasing the risk of heart disease and inflammation.

Myths about Fat

Myth 1: Eating fat makes you fat.

This simplistic view has been debunked. Weight gain occurs when caloric intake exceeds caloric expenditure, regardless of whether those calories come from fat, protein, or carbohydrates. In fact, fat is more satiating than carbohydrates, meaning it can help reduce overeating and support weight management.

Myth 2: Low-fat diets are healthier.

Low-fat diets were once considered the gold standard for health, but they often lead to increased consumption of processed carbohydrates and sugars. Studies now show that diets rich in healthy fats are more effective at reducing heart disease risk, managing diabetes, and supporting weight loss.

Myth 3: All saturated fats are bad.

While saturated fats should be consumed in moderation, they are not inherently harmful. The context matters—saturated fats from whole foods like grass-fed beef and coconut oil are less concerning than those from processed junk food.

Myth 4: Cholesterol in food equals high cholesterol in blood.

For decades, dietary cholesterol (from foods like eggs) was vilified. However, research has shown that dietary cholesterol has little impact on blood cholesterol levels for most people. The real culprits are trans fats and excessive sugar intake.

Emotional and Cultural Connections to Fat

Our relationship with fat isn't just biological—it's deeply emotional and cultural. For decades, consumers have been bombarded with messages equating fat consumption with guilt and failure. "Low-fat" labels became a moral badge of health-consciousness, even as the products bearing them were packed with sugar and artificial ingredients.

Cultural cuisines provide a stark contrast. Mediterranean diets, rich in olive oil, nuts, and fish, have long been celebrated for their health benefits. Similarly, traditional diets in regions like Okinawa and Sardinia feature healthy fats as staples, contributing to their populations' longevity. These examples remind us that fats can be part of a healthy, vibrant way of eating when consumed in balance.

The Role of Healthy Fats in the Body

1. Brain health

The brain is nearly 60 percent fat, and healthy fats are critical for its function. Omega-3 fatty acids, in particular, are essential for cognitive development, memory, and mood regulation. Low omega-3 intake has been linked to depression, anxiety, and cognitive decline.

2. Heart health

Contrary to outdated beliefs, many fats protect the heart. Monounsaturated and polyunsaturated fats help reduce inflammation and lower the risk of heart disease. Omega-3s have been shown to reduce triglycerides, prevent arrhythmias, and decrease blood pressure.

3. Nutrient absorption

Fat-soluble vitamins (A, D, E, and K) require dietary fat for absorption. Without enough fat in the diet, these essential nutrients cannot be properly utilized by the body.

4. Energy source

Fats are a dense source of energy, providing 9 calories per gram—more than double the energy of carbohydrates or proteins. This makes fats an important fuel source, especially during prolonged physical activity or when carbohydrate intake is limited.

Practical Tips for Incorporating Healthy Fats

1. Choose quality over quantity.

Opt for whole, unprocessed sources of fat, like avocados, nuts, seeds, and fatty fish. Avoid processed snacks and fried foods that contain trans fats or hydrogenated oils.

2. Embrace olive oil.

Extra virgin olive oil is a cornerstone of the Mediterranean diet, and one of the healthiest fats you can consume. Use it for cooking, dressings, and dips.

3. Snack smart.

Instead of reaching for chips or sugary snacks, try a handful of almonds, walnuts, or pumpkin seeds. These snacks are nutrient-dense and satisfying.

4. Cook with healthy fats.

Use coconut oil or ghee for high-heat cooking, and save olive oil for low-heat applications or as a finishing touch.

5. Add fat to every meal.

Incorporating healthy fats into every meal can help keep you full and stabilize blood sugar levels. Add avocado to your breakfast, drizzle olive oil on your salad, or enjoy a piece of dark chocolate as a treat.

The Future of Fats

As our understanding of fats continues to evolve, the narrative is shifting from fear to appreciation. Research highlights the importance of distinguishing between different types of fats and prioritizing quality over quantity. While the damage done by the low-fat craze won't be undone overnight, a growing body of evidence is restoring fats to their rightful place in a balanced diet.

Ultimately, the key is balance. Healthy fats, consumed in moderation, can nourish the body, support long-term health, and even enhance our enjoyment of food. It's time to move beyond outdated myths and embrace a more nuanced approach to dietary fat—one that celebrates its role in a vibrant, healthy lifestyle.

The story of fat is one of redemption. From decades of vilification to its modern renaissance, fat has proven itself to be far more than the villain it was once made out to be. By understanding the facts and rejecting the fiction, we can reclaim fat as a powerful ally in our pursuit of health and well-being.

CHAPTER

5

The Role of Additives
and Preservatives

Modern food is a chemical cocktail. The brightly colored cereal boxes lining grocery store aisles, the soft texture of packaged bread, and the long shelf life of processed snacks are all made possible by additives and preservatives. These chemical compounds enhance flavor, extend freshness, and ensure visual appeal. However, these innovations come at a significant cost: the potential toll on human health.

While food additives are often marketed as harmless, or even essential, the reality is more complex. Some additives are benign, or naturally derived, but others are synthetic compounds that have sparked debates and scientific scrutiny for decades. In this chapter, we will dive into the history, science, myths, and truths behind food additives and preservatives. By examining their purposes, the health risks they may pose, and the controversies surrounding them, you'll gain a clearer understanding of what's really in your food—and why it matters.

The Rise of Additives in the Food Industry

The use of additives and preservatives in food is not new. Ancient civilizations used salt, honey, and vinegar to preserve meats and fruits, leveraging natural methods to extend food's shelf life. However, the industrial revolution in the nineteenth century marked a turning point. As urban populations grew and transportation systems improved, the demand for long-lasting, easily transportable food increased. This spurred the creation of synthetic additives, revolutionizing the way food was produced, stored, and consumed.

Fast-forward to the twentieth century, and the food industry exploded with new products. Supermarkets replaced local markets, and packaged, processed foods became the norm. To meet consumer demands for convenience, manufacturers began adding substances like artificial colors, flavors, and preservatives to their products. These additives not only extended shelf life but also made food visually appealing and consistently flavorful.

However, the rapid expansion of chemical use in food production raised questions about safety. Were these additives truly necessary? Could they harm human health in the long term? While regulatory agencies like the US Food and Drug Administration (FDA) and the European Food Safety Authority (EFSA) were established to monitor food safety, some critics argue that regulations lag behind the pace of scientific discovery.

The Most Common Additives and Their Functions

Food additives serve various purposes. Here's a breakdown of the most common types and their intended benefits:

1. Preservatives

Purpose: Prevent spoilage caused by microorganisms like bacteria, yeast, and mold.

Examples: Sodium nitrite, sodium benzoate, and potassium sorbate.

Controversies: Some preservatives, like sodium nitrite, are linked to the formation of carcinogenic compounds during cooking.

2. Artificial colors

Purpose: Enhance or restore the color of food to make it more visually appealing. Examples: Yellow 5, Red 40, and Blue 1.
Health concerns: Studies suggest links between artificial dyes and hyperactivity in children, as well as potential allergic reactions.

3. Artificial flavors

Purpose: Mimic natural flavors to create consistent taste profiles in processed foods.

Examples: Vanillin, artificial strawberry flavoring.
Debate: The long-term effects of synthetic flavor compounds are still being studied.

4. Emulsifiers and stabilizers

Purpose: Improve texture and consistency in products like ice cream, salad dressings, and baked goods.

Examples: Lecithin, carrageenan, and xanthan gum.

Concerns: Some additives, like carrageenan, have been associated with gastrointestinal inflammation.

5. Sweeteners

Purpose: Provide sweetness without the calories of sugar. Examples: Aspartame, saccharin, and sucralose.
Health risks: Aspartame, in particular, has been a lightning rod for controversy, with conflicting studies on its potential carcinogenicity.

Truths about Food Additives

Truth 1: They are heavily regulated (in most countries).

Food additives undergo rigorous testing before being approved for use. Regulatory agencies establish acceptable daily intake (ADI) levels to minimize risks. However, critics argue that these tests often rely on animal studies and may not accurately predict human responses over a lifetime of exposure.

Truth 2: Not all additives are synthetic.

Many additives are derived from natural sources. For example, lecithin, an emulsifier, comes from soybeans or egg yolks, and citric acid is derived from citrus fruits.

Truth 3: Additives can help prevent foodborne illness.

Preservatives like sodium benzoate inhibit the growth of harmful bacteria such as *Clostridium botulinum*, which causes botulism—a potentially fatal condition.

Myths Surrounding Additives

Myth 1: All additives are harmful.

Not all additives are inherently dangerous. Some, like ascorbic acid (vitamin C) and tocopherols (vitamin E), are added to prevent oxidation and are beneficial to health.

Myth 2: Natural additives are always better than synthetic ones.

Natural additives can also pose risks. For example, some people are allergic to annatto, a natural coloring agent derived from seeds. Additionally, natural additives can be less stable and require higher concentrations to achieve the same effect as synthetic alternatives.

Myth 3: Foods without additives are safer.

While reducing processed food consumption is generally healthy, the absence of additives does not guarantee safety. Fresh produce, for instance, can harbor pathogens if not handled properly.

The Dark Side of Additives

Hyperactivity and artificial dyes

Artificial food colorings, particularly Yellow 5 and Red 40, have been linked to behavioral issues in children. A landmark study in 2007 by the University of Southampton found that certain artificial dyes exacerbated hyperactivity in children, leading some countries to require warning labels on products containing these additives.

Cancer and preservatives

Nitrates and nitrites, commonly found in processed meats like bacon and hot dogs, can transform into nitrosamines when exposed to high heat. Nitrosamines are classified as probable carcinogens by the International Agency for Research on Cancer (IARC).

Despite this, processed meats *remain* a staple in many diets worldwide.

The hidden sugar trap

Artificial sweeteners, often marketed as "diet-friendly," come with their own set of risks. Research has linked high aspartame consumption to potential disruptions in gut microbiota, and even an increased risk of metabolic disorders.

The emotional toll of hidden additives

For many consumers, the discovery of harmful additives in everyday foods can feel like a betrayal. Imagine a parent carefully selecting snacks for their child, only to learn later that the brightly colored candies contain dyes associated with hyperactivity. Similarly, individuals seeking to lose weight may turn to "sugar-free" products, unaware of the potential risks posed by artificial sweeteners.

This sense of deception is compounded by the marketing tactics employed by food companies. Terms like "natural," "organic," and "healthy" can be misleading, giving consumers a false sense of security.

Taking Control: How to Avoid Harmful Additives

1. Read labels carefully.

Familiarize yourself with common additives and their potential effects. Apps and online databases can help decode complex ingredient lists.

2. Choose whole foods.

Opt for minimally processed foods like fresh fruits, vegetables, whole grains, and lean proteins.

3. Support transparent brands.

Look for companies that prioritize clean labeling and disclose all ingredients.

4. Cook at home.

Preparing meals from scratch allows you to control what goes into your food.

5. Advocate for stronger regulations.

Support policies that require clearer labeling and stricter testing of food additives.

The Future of Food Additives

Advances in food science are paving the way for safer, more sustainable additives. Researchers are exploring plant-based preservatives and natural antimicrobials to replace synthetic chemicals. Innovations in biotechnology may also allow for the creation of additives that are indistinguishable from their natural counterparts, minimizing health risks.

CHAPTER

6

The Fast-Food Epidemic

Fast food is more than a meal—it's a cultural phenomenon. From iconic golden arches to catchy jingles promising "I'm lovin' it," fast food is woven into the fabric of daily life in America. What began as a novelty in the mid-twentieth century has transformed into an omnipresent force shaping diets, health, and even the environment. But behind the convenience and low price lies a dark reality: Fast food is engineered not just to satisfy but to hook you. The cost? Far greater than the dollar menu suggests.

The Allure of Fast Food

Cheap, quick, and tasty: These are the promises that fast food delivers on, which makes it almost irresistible. For busy families, overworked professionals, or students on a budget, fast food feels like a lifeline. But this perceived convenience has been meticulously designed to appeal to your senses and override your better judgment.

Fast food relies on the bliss point. The trifecta of precisely combined sugar, salt, and fat lights up the brain's reward centers, flooding you with dopamine, the chemical associated with pleasure. The problem? This artificial stimulation creates a cycle of cravings that can be as addictive as drugs. Studies have shown that the brain's response to a cheeseburger or milkshake mimics its reaction to cocaine or nicotine.

Moreover, fast-food restaurants strategically design their menus and promotions to encourage overconsumption. Supersizing, combo deals, and limited-time offers aren't just marketing tactics—they are psychological traps designed to make you buy and eat more than you need.

A Growing Health Crisis

The convenience of fast food comes at a steep cost to your health. In the United States, obesity rates have more than tripled since the 1970s, coinciding with the rise of fast-food chains. According to the Centers for Disease Control and Prevention (CDC), nearly 42% of American adults are obese, and fast food plays a significant role in this epidemic.

Fast food is calorie-dense but nutrient-poor, a combination that sets the stage for weight gain and chronic health conditions. Consider this: A large fast-food meal can contain more calories, sugar, and sodium than an adult should consume in an entire day. For example, a Big Mac, large fries, and soda total nearly 1,300 calories, over 1,300 milligrams of sodium, and 55 grams of sugar—yet they provide little in the way of fiber, vitamins, or other essential nutrients.

The effects extend far beyond weight gain. Regular consumption of fast food has been linked to the following:

Type 2 diabetes. The excessive sugar and refined carbohydrates in fast food spike blood sugar levels, increasing insulin resistance over time.

Heart disease. High levels of trans fats and sodium elevate cholesterol and blood pressure, leading to cardiovascular problems.

Digestive disorders. Preservatives and artificial additives can disrupt gut health, contributing to bloating, constipation, and other issues.

Mental health problems. Emerging research suggests a connection between poor diet quality and depression, anxiety, and cognitive decline.

One shocking study found that people who eat fast food more than four times a week have an 80% higher risk of developing type 2 diabetes. Another revealed that the average fast-food consumer ingests up to twenty pounds of french fries annually. These staggering statistics highlight the long-term consequences of choosing convenience over health.

The Emotional Toll of Fast Food

Fast food doesn't just affect your physical health—it also takes a toll on your emotions. Many people develop a love-hate relationship with it. They turn to fast food for comfort during stressful times, only to feel guilt and shame afterward. This cycle of emotional eating is reinforced by the addictive qualities of fast food, creating a feedback loop that's difficult to break.

Take, for example, the story of Jamie, a single mother working two jobs. With little time to cook, she relies on fast food to feed her two children. While it saves time and money, Jamie notices her kids becoming sluggish, gaining weight, and struggling with focus in school. She feels guilty but sees no way out. "It's a vicious cycle," she says. "Fast food feels like the only option, but I know it's hurting my family."

For many, fast food represents a quick fix that ultimately exacerbates deeper issues. Its affordability and ubiquity mask the long-term damage it can cause—not just to individuals but to families and communities as well.

The Environmental Cost of Fast Food

The fast-food epidemic isn't just a public health crisis—it's an environmental one too. From factory farming to excessive packaging, the industry leaves a massive ecological footprint.

1. Factory farming and deforestation

Fast food relies heavily on factory-farmed meat, which contributes to deforestation, greenhouse gas emissions, and water pollution. For example, the production of beef for a single burger requires approximately 660 gallons of water. Moreover, the demand for cheap meat drives deforestation in regions like the Amazon rainforest, where land is cleared for cattle grazing.

2. Packaging waste

Fast-food meals generate enormous amounts of single-use packaging, much of which ends up in landfills or as litter. According to the Environmental Protection Agency (EPA), fast-food packaging accounts for a significant portion of urban waste, contributing to pollution and harm to wildlife.

3. Energy and resources

The energy-intensive processes of producing, transporting, and cooking fast food contribute to climate change. A study by the Natural Resources Defense Council (NRDC) found that the fast-food industry emits millions of tons of carbon dioxide annually, making it a major contributor to global warming.

Marketing to the Vulnerable

Fast-food companies are masters of manipulation, targeting their marketing efforts at vulnerable populations, including children, low-income families, and communities of color. Research shows that fast-food chains disproportionately advertise unhealthy options in minority neighborhoods, where access to fresh, affordable food is often limited.

Children are particularly susceptible to fast-food marketing. Brightly colored mascots, toys in kids' meals, and TV commercials create lifelong brand loyalty. Studies reveal that children as young as three can recognize fast-food logos and associate them with happiness. This early exposure contributes to unhealthy eating habits that persist into adulthood.

Low-income families face a unique dilemma. With limited budgets and tight schedules, fast food often feels like the only viable option. But this accessibility is by design. Many fast-food chains strategically place locations near schools, public housing, and bus stops, ensuring their products remain a constant presence in vulnerable communities.

Breaking Free from the Fast-Food Trap

Escaping the fast-food trap doesn't mean giving up convenience—it means redefining it.

Here are practical steps to reduce your reliance on fast food without sacrificing time or flavor:

1. Practice meal prep and planning.

Dedicate a few hours each week to preparing simple, healthy meals that you can reheat. Batch-cooking staples like soups, stir-fries, and grain bowls makes it easy to grab a nutritious option on busy days.

2. Choose healthier fast-food options.

If you must eat fast food, look for items with grilled proteins, fresh vegetables, and whole grains. Many chains now offer healthier options, though it's crucial to read the fine print.

3. Support local alternatives.

Seek out local delis, salad bars, or food trucks that prioritize fresh, wholesome ingredients. These alternatives are often just as convenient, and far more nutritious.

4. Educate yourself and your family.

Teach your children about the importance of balanced eating. Involve them in grocery shopping and cooking to foster a positive relationship with food.

A Call for Change

The fast-food epidemic is not solely the result of individual choices—it's a systemic issue rooted in corporate greed, government policies, and societal norms. Addressing it requires collective action, from advocating for stricter food labeling laws to supporting policies that promote food equity.

As consumers, we have power. Every dollar spent on fresh, wholesome food is a vote against the fast-food industry's exploitative practices. By making mindful choices, we can begin to dismantle the fast-food empire and build a healthier future.

Fast food may be a part of our culture, but it doesn't have to define our diets. The first step to change is awareness, and with that awareness comes the power to take back control of our health and our lives.

CHAPTER

7

The Silent Killer: Sodium Overload

Salt has long been a staple of human civilization. It was once so valuable that it was used as currency, and its ability to preserve food revolutionized trade and survival. However, in today's world, salt is no longer a rarity; instead, it has become a dietary hazard. Americans, on average, consume more than double the recommended daily intake of sodium, with devastating consequences. The problem isn't just the salt you sprinkle on your food—it's the hidden sodium lurking in processed and restaurant meals, quietly wreaking havoc on your health.

In this chapter, we will uncover the truth about sodium overload, dispel common myths about salt, and explore practical ways to protect yourself and your loved ones from its harmful effects.

The Essential Role of Salt

Let's begin with the basics: Salt, or sodium chloride, is essential for life. Sodium helps regulate fluid balance, supports nerve function, and assists muscle contractions.

Without it, the human body cannot function. The recommended daily intake of sodium for adults is around 2,300 milligrams (about one teaspoon of salt), with an ideal limit of 1,500 milligrams for those with high blood pressure or other risk factors.

But herein lies the paradox: While some sodium is necessary, too much can be deadly. Consuming excessive amounts over time can lead to a host of health issues, turning this vital nutrient into a silent killer.

How Sodium Affects Your Body

When you consume too much sodium, your body retains excess water to dilute it. This additional fluid increases blood volume, forcing your heart to work harder and raising your blood pressure. Over time, this extra strain damages blood vessels, contributes to plaque buildup, and increases the risk of heart disease and stroke.

Here's how sodium wreaks havoc with your health:

Hypertension (high blood pressure). Excess sodium is a leading cause of hypertension, a condition that affects nearly half of all American adults. Often called the silent killer, hypertension shows no symptoms until it causes serious complications like heart attacks or strokes.

Kidney damage. Your kidneys play a critical role in filtering excess sodium from your blood. Chronic overconsumption can overwork the kidneys, leading to reduced function or kidney disease.

Osteoporosis. High sodium intake can cause calcium to be excreted in urine, weakening bones over time and increasing the risk of osteoporosis.

Fluid retention and bloating. Consuming too much sodium can lead to uncomfortable water retention, causing swelling in the hands, feet, and face.

The Hidden Sodium Problem

Most people think of salty snacks like chips or pretzels when they hear the word "sodium," but the real danger lies in the sodium you can't taste.

Processed foods and restaurant meals are often loaded with hidden sodium to enhance flavor, preserve shelf life, and improve texture.

Consider these everyday culprits:

Bread and rolls. A single slice of bread can contain up to 200 milligrams of sodium, and the average sandwich easily exceeds 500 milligrams before any condiments are added.

Canned soups. Many canned soups contain over 900 milligrams of sodium per serving—nearly half the daily recommended limit in just one bowl.

Deli meats. Processed meats like ham, turkey, and salami are loaded with sodium, with some varieties packing 1,000 milligrams or more per serving.

Condiments. Ketchup, soy sauce, salad dressings, and pickles are sodium bombs in disguise. A single tablespoon of soy sauce can deliver over 1,000 milligrams of sodium.

Frozen meals. Many frozen dinners are marketed as "healthy" but contain 700–1,500 milligrams of sodium per serving.

Even foods that don't taste salty, such as breakfast cereals or desserts, can contain surprising amounts of sodium. Manufacturers often use sodium-based additives like baking soda, monosodium glutamate (MSG), and sodium nitrate to enhance flavor or extend shelf life.

The Numbers Don't Lie

The average American consumes 3,400 milligrams of sodium per day, far exceeding the recommended limit.

Let's put this into perspective:

- One slice of pizza can have up to 760 milligrams of sodium.
- A fast-food burger with fries can total over 2,000 milligrams of sodium.
- A single serving of ramen noodles contains a staggering 1,760 milligrams of sodium—nearly your entire daily allowance in one meal.

These numbers reveal how easy it is to consume excessive sodium without realizing it.

Myths about Salt

Despite overwhelming evidence of sodium's harmful effects, several myths persist that downplay its dangers. Let's debunk them.

Myth 1: As long as you don't add salt to your food, you're fine.

The saltshaker is not the primary source of sodium in most diets. Processed and restaurant foods account for over 70% of sodium intake in the average American diet.

Myth 2: If you don't have high blood pressure, you don't need to worry.

Even if you don't have hypertension now, excessive sodium intake increases your risk over time. High sodium levels can also harm your heart, kidneys, and bones, regardless of your blood pressure.

Myth 3: Sea salt and Himalayan salt are healthier.

These trendy salts contain trace minerals but have nearly the same sodium content as regular table salt. They are not a healthier alternative when consumed in excess.

Myth 4: You need more salt if you exercise a lot."

While athletes may lose sodium through sweat, the average person doesn't need extra salt to compensate for physical activity.

Emotional Narratives: The Human Toll

Behind the statistics are real stories of lives impacted by sodium overload. Consider Maria, a fifty-year-old nurse who thought her diet was "pretty healthy." She rarely added salt to her meals and avoided junk food, yet she suffered a stroke at age forty-nine. The culprit? Her daily "healthy" lunch of canned soup and deli turkey wraps, which added up to 2,800 milligrams of sodium per day.

Then there's David, a thirty-five-year-old father of two who relied on frozen meals and fast food to save time. When he was diagnosed with hypertension, he was shocked. "I didn't even realize I was eating so much salt," he says. "It was hidden in everything I thought was convenient."

These stories highlight how sodium sneaks into our diets, causing damage long before symptoms appear.

Practical Tips to Reduce Sodium in Your Food

Reducing sodium doesn't mean sacrificing flavor. With small changes, you can significantly cut your intake while still enjoying delicious meals.

1. Read labels.

Look for foods labeled "low sodium," "reduced sodium," or "no added salt." Aim for products with less than 140 milligrams of sodium per serving.

2. Cook at home.

Homemade meals give you control over the amount of salt that goes into your food. Use fresh herbs, spices, garlic, or lemon juice to enhance flavor naturally.

3. Rinse canned foods.

If you must use canned beans or vegetables, rinse them under cold water to remove excess sodium.

4. Choose fresh or frozen.

Opt for fresh or frozen fruits and vegetables instead of canned or preseasoned options.

5. Limit condiments. Use low-sodium versions of ketchup, soy sauce, and salad dressings, or make your own at home.

6. Be mindful at restaurants. Request your meal with no added salt, and avoid high-sodium menu items like soups and sauces.

7. Watch portion sizes. Eating smaller portions can reduce your overall sodium intake without depriving yourself of your favorite foods.

A Call for Awareness and Action

The sodium crisis isn't just an individual problem—it's a systemic one. Food manufacturers and restaurants prioritize profit over public health, using sodium as a cheap way to enhance flavor and extend shelf life. Advocacy for clearer food labeling and stricter regulations on sodium content is essential to combat this silent killer.

As consumers, we can drive change by voting with our wallets. Supporting brands and restaurants that prioritize low-sodium options sends a powerful message to the industry. Together, we can demand a food system that values health over convenience.

Final Thoughts

Salt may be essential, but its overuse is deadly. By becoming aware of hidden sodium, debunking myths, and making informed choices, you can protect yourself from the silent killer lurking in your diet.

Remember, small changes add up: every lower-sodium meal you choose is a step toward better health.

Your life—and the lives of those you care about—is worth the effort. The journey to better health starts with awareness and a commitment to change.

CHAPTER

8

Food Deserts and Accessibility

Imagine living in a neighborhood where the nearest grocery store is miles away, but fast food restaurants and convenience stores are within walking distance. Fresh fruits and vegetables are a rarity, while processed, high-calorie, low-nutrient options dominate the shelves.

This is the daily reality for millions of Americans living in food deserts—areas where access to affordable, nutritious food is limited or nonexistent.

Food deserts are not just a symptom of poverty—they are a stark reminder of systemic inequities embedded in America's food system. These deserts perpetuate cycles of poor health, economic instability, and social inequality, disproportionately affecting low-income families and communities of color.

This chapter takes an in-depth look at the causes, consequences, and potential solutions for food deserts. By understanding the barriers to healthy eating and the grassroots efforts aimed at addressing them, we can advocate for a more equitable food system and help break the chains of food insecurity.

Defining Food Deserts

The term "food desert" might evoke images of barren, lifeless landscapes, but the reality is far more insidious. Food deserts exist in both urban and rural areas, defined by their lack of access to full-service grocery stores or supermarkets that provide fresh, affordable, and nutritious food.

The United States Department of Agriculture (USDA) considers an area a food desert if:

- Urban residents must travel more than one mile to reach a grocery store.
- Rural residents must travel more than ten miles to access fresh produce and other essentials.

While distance is a critical factor, food deserts are also shaped by economic barriers, such as low incomes, limited transportation options, and the higher cost of healthier options. These factors converge to create an environment where residents face significant challenges in accessing nutritious meals.

The Scope of the Problem

The statistics surrounding food deserts are staggering:

Over 19 million Americans live in food deserts, according to the USDA.

Roughly 39.5 million people live in low-income neighborhoods with limited supermarket access.

African American and Latino communities are disproportionately affected, with a 70% higher likelihood of living in food deserts compared to white communities.

These figures underscore how systemic inequities—rooted in socioeconomic disparities, racial segregation, and urban planning decisions—have shaped the geography of food deserts in America.

The Roots of Food Deserts

Food deserts didn't emerge overnight; they are the result of decades of systemic neglect and discriminatory practices. Here are some of the key factors that have contributed to their development:

- Urban decline and suburbanization

In the mid-twentieth century, urban areas experienced significant economic decline as middle-class families moved to the suburbs. Supermarkets followed, leaving behind low-income urban neighborhoods with dwindling access to fresh food.

- Racial segregation

Redlining—a discriminatory practice where banks refused loans to predominantly Black neighborhoods—prevented communities of color from accumulating wealth and accessing resources, including grocery stores. The legacy of redlining persists today, with many historically redlined areas now classified as food deserts.

- Economic inequality

Low-income neighborhoods are less profitable for large grocery chains due to lesser spending power and higher operational costs. As a result, these areas are underserved by retailers, creating a void filled by fast-food outlets and convenience stores.

- Transportation barriers

Many residents of food deserts lack access to reliable transportation, making it difficult to travel to grocery stores outside their neighborhoods. Public transit options are often limited or nonexistent in rural areas, compounding the problem.

Consequences of Food Deserts

The impact of living in a food desert extends far beyond an empty fridge. It affects nearly every aspect of life, from health to education to economic opportunity.

- Health disparities

Food deserts contribute to alarming health disparities, including:

Obesity. The reliance on calorie-dense, nutrient-poor foods increases the risk of obesity.

Diabetes. Limited access to fresh fruits and vegetables exacerbates the prevalence of type 2 diabetes.

Heart disease. Diets high in sodium, sugar, and unhealthy fats contribute to cardiovascular problems.

Malnutrition. Ironically, many residents of food deserts suffer from malnutrition despite consuming high-calorie diets, as processed foods lack essential nutrients.

- Economic struggles

Poor health resulting from inadequate diets leads to higher medical bills, missed workdays, and reduced productivity, perpetuating cycles of poverty.

- Educational impact

Children in food deserts are more likely to experience developmental delays, learning difficulties, and behavioral problems due to poor nutrition. Hunger and malnutrition impair their ability to focus in school, limiting future opportunities.

- Social isolation

The absence of grocery stores and fresh food options contributes to feelings of neglect and marginalization, reinforcing systemic inequalities and limiting community cohesion.

The Role of Fast Food Restaurants and Convenience Stores

In the absence of grocery stores, residents of food deserts often turn to fast food and convenience stores for sustenance. These outlets prioritize profit over nutrition, offering cheap, processed foods loaded with calories, sugar, and unhealthy fats.

For example:

A fast-food meal may cost less than $5, but it provides minimal nutritional value.

Convenience store snacks like chips and soda are often the only available options, perpetuating poor dietary habits.

While these choices are understandable given the circumstances, they come at a heavy cost to public health.

Dispelling Myths about Food Deserts

Several misconceptions about food deserts must be addressed:

Myth 1: People in food deserts just need to make better choices.

Truth: When access to fresh food is limited, the ability to make healthy choices is severely constrained. It's not about willpower—it's about systemic barriers.

Myth: Fast food is cheaper than cooking at home.

Truth: While fast food may seem cheaper up front, cooking in bulk with fresh ingredients is often more cost-effective in the long run. However, the up-front cost and lack of access to fresh ingredients make this option unattainable for many in food deserts.

Myth 3: Food deserts exist only in cities.

Truth: Rural areas are also affected by food deserts, often to an even greater extent due to transportation barriers and low population density.

Stories from the Front Lines

The human stories behind food deserts reveal the emotional toll they take on families and communities.

Maria's Struggle

A single mother in Detroit, Maria works two jobs to support her three children. The nearest grocery store is five miles away, but without a car, she relies on the corner store for groceries. Her kids often eat instant noodles and chips, a diet she knows is unhealthy but feels powerless to change. "I want to give my kids better, but how can I do that when this is all I have?" she asks.

James's Fight for Change

In a rural Kentucky town, James, a retired farmer, has started a community garden to combat the lack of fresh produce. "We can't wait for supermarkets to come to us," he says. "We have to take matters into our own hands."

These stories highlight the resilience of those living in food deserts and the urgency of addressing this issue.

Grassroots Efforts to Combat Food Deserts

Despite the challenges, there are inspiring initiatives across the country aimed at tackling food deserts:

1. Community gardens: Neighborhoods are turning vacant lots into thriving gardens that provide fresh produce and foster a sense of community.

2. Mobile markets: Nonprofits like Fresh Moves bring fresh fruits and vegetables to underserved areas using retrofitted buses or trucks.

3. Food co-ops: Local co-ops allow communities to pool resources and create their own grocery stores, prioritizing affordability and nutrition.

4. Policy advocacy: Organizations like the Food Trust work to influence policies that incentivize grocery stores to open in food deserts and improve food access.

How You Can Make a Difference

Addressing food deserts requires collective action. Here's how you can contribute:

1. Support local farmers' markets and community gardens.

2. Volunteer with or donate to organizations tackling food insecurity.

3. Advocate for policies that promote food equity, such as subsidies for grocery stores in underserved areas.

4. Raise awareness about food deserts in your community to drive systemic change.

A Vision for a More Equitable Food System

Food deserts are a symptom of deeper systemic issues, but they are not an unsolvable problem. With innovation, collaboration, and policy reform, we can reimagine a food system that prioritizes health and equity over profit.

Access to fresh, nutritious food is not a privilege—it's a basic human right. By working together, we can ensure that no one has to live in a food desert and every family has the opportunity to thrive.

9

Taking Back Control
of Your Health

The modern food landscape often feels like an unrelenting tide of convenience, marketing, and misinformation. Processed foods, fast meals, and hidden ingredients dominate our plates, making it easy to lose control over what we eat and, ultimately, our health. But reclaiming your well-being doesn't require drastic overhauls or unattainable goals. It begins with small, intentional changes that build over time.

This chapter is a guide to taking back control of your health—not just for personal benefit but also as part of a broader movement to demand a food system that prioritizes people over profits. By understanding the truths behind our food choices and making conscious decisions, we can break free from unhealthy cycles and redefine our relationship with food.

The Struggle for Control

Why does it feel so difficult to make healthy choices? The food industry has spent billions of dollars engineering convenience and addiction into our diets. Processed foods are designed to hit the bliss point so we would keep coming back for more. Marketing reinforces these choices, presenting fast food and snacks as quick fixes for busy lives.

But the consequences are undeniable: rising rates of obesity, diabetes, heart disease, and other chronic conditions. This is not a failure of individual willpower—it's the result of a system that profits from unhealthy habits. Reclaiming control means understanding the forces at play and taking deliberate steps to counter them.

The Power of Small Changes

When faced with the enormity of health challenges, it's easy to feel overwhelmed. But lasting change rarely happens overnight. Instead, it begins with small, manageable shifts in your daily routine.

1. Start with awareness.

Read labels. The first step is understanding what you're consuming. Food labels can be misleading, with hidden sugars, sodium, and artificial ingredients. Look beyond the marketing and examine the ingredients list.

Track your eating habits. Keep a food journal for a week. Note what you eat, when, and how it makes you feel. Patterns will emerge, revealing areas for improvement.

2. Cook at home.

Home-cooked meals give you control over ingredients, portion sizes, and flavors.

Start simple. Replace one processed meal a week with a homemade dish. Gradually increase this as you grow more comfortable in the kitchen.

Experiment with spices, herbs, and fresh ingredients to make meals flavorful without relying on added sugars or salts.

3. Focus on whole, unprocessed foods.

Aim for a diet rich in fruits, vegetables, whole grains, lean proteins, and healthy fats.

Avoid foods with long ingredient lists or those you can't pronounce—these are often highly processed.

4.   Hydrate mindfully.

Sugary drinks are a hidden source of calories and sugar. Replace sodas and energy drinks with water, herbal teas, or infused water.

Keep a reusable water bottle with you to encourage consistent hydration.

Meal Planning: A Game Changer

One of the most effective tools for taking control of your health is meal planning. It removes the guesswork from daily eating, reduces reliance on convenience foods, and saves both time and money.

Steps to Successful Meal Planning

1.   Assess your week.

Consider your schedule, including work, family commitments, and social events. Plan meals that fit your lifestyle.

2.   Choose recipes.

Select a mix of simple, nutritious recipes that you enjoy. Include a variety of proteins, vegetables, and grains for balanced meals.

3.   Make a shopping list.

Write down all the ingredients you need and stick to your list at the grocery store. This helps avoid impulse purchases.

4.   Prep ahead.

Spend a few hours each week chopping vegetables, cooking grains, or preparing sauces. This makes assembling meals during the week faster and easier.

Batch Cooking and Freezing

Cooking in bulk is a time-saving strategy that ensures you always have healthy options on hand. Freeze individual portions of soups, stews, or casseroles for quick meals.

Breaking Free from Myths

The journey to better health is often clouded by myths and misconceptions that can derail progress. Let's debunk some of the most common ones:

Myth: Healthy eating is expensive.

While some organic or specialty products can be pricey, healthy eating doesn't have to break the bank. Buying seasonal produce, shopping at local farmers' markets, and cooking at home can save money. Beans, lentils, rice, and frozen vegetables are budget-friendly staples.

Myth: People don't have time to eat healthily.

Time constraints are a valid concern, but meal prepping and batch cooking can help. Even a quick fifteen-minute stir-fry with fresh vegetables and lean protein is a healthier option than fast food.

Myth: Fat is bad for you.

Not all fats are created equal. Healthy fats from sources like avocados, nuts, seeds, and olive oil are essential for brain function, hormone production, and overall health.

Myth: Skipping meals will help you lose weight.

Skipping meals can lead to overeating later and disrupt your metabolism. Focus on balanced, consistent meals to fuel your body.

Advocating for a Better Food System

Taking control of your health isn't just about individual choices—it's about challenging the broader system that shapes our food environment. Advocacy can take many forms, from supporting local farmers to pushing for policy changes that make nutritious food accessible to everyone.

Grassroots Advocacy

Support farmers' markets. Buying directly from farmers supports local agriculture and ensures you're getting fresh, seasonal produce.

Volunteer at food banks. Help provide healthy food options to those in need.

Policy Change

Advocate for legislation that addresses food deserts, supports nutrition education, and regulates harmful food marketing practices.

Push for transparency in food labeling to empower consumers.

Demanding Accountability

Hold corporations accountable for prioritizing profits over public health. Support brands and businesses that value sustainability, transparency, and nutrition.

Emotional Barriers to Change

Taking back control of your health is not just a physical journey—it's an emotional one. Many people have deep-seated relationships with food that are tied to comfort, tradition, or even trauma. Recognizing and addressing these emotional barriers is crucial for lasting change.

Food as comfort. It's common to turn to food for emotional support. Identifying triggers and finding alternative coping mechanisms, like exercise or journaling, can help break this cycle.

Cultural traditions. Many family recipes are high in salt, sugar, or fat. Rather than abandoning these traditions, look for ways to modify them to be healthier without losing their essence.

Shame and guilt. Avoid the all-or-nothing mindset. One unhealthy meal doesn't undo progress. Focus on consistency rather than perfection.

Stories of Transformation

Real-life stories can inspire and motivate change. Consider Sarah, a forty-two-year-old mother of two who felt overwhelmed by the idea of overhauling her diet. She started small by replacing her morning sugary cereal with oatmeal and fresh fruit. Over time, she incorporated more vegetables into her meals and began cooking at home. "I never thought I could stick with it," she says, "but now I feel stronger and more in control than ever."

Then there's Marcus, a fifty-eight-year-old truck driver who struggled with hypertension and obesity. After attending a community nutrition class, he started packing healthy snacks like nuts, fruits, and homemade sandwiches for his long hauls. "I've lost thirty pounds," he says. "But more importantly, I've gained confidence in my ability to take care of myself."

The Ripple Effect

When one person takes control of their health, the benefits extend far beyond the individual. Families adopt healthier habits, communities demand better food options, and industries feel the pressure to change.

By prioritizing your health, you're not just improving your life—you're contributing to a movement that challenges the status quo and advocates for a food system that values well-being over profit.

FINAL THOUGHTS

Empower Yourself

Taking back control of your health is a journey, not a destination. It's about making informed decisions, embracing progress over perfection, and finding joy in nourishing your body.

Remember, every small change matters. Each home-cooked meal, every label read, and every step toward a healthier lifestyle brings you closer to reclaiming your well-being. And as you transform your relationship with food, you will inspire others to do the same, creating a ripple effect of positive change in your community and beyond.

Your health is your greatest asset. Take it back—one mindful choice at a time.

REFERENCES

Centers for Disease Control and Prevention. (2022). "Obesity and Overweight." https://www.cdc.gov/obesity/data/adult.html

Food and Drug Administration. (2020). "Food Additives and Ingredients." https://www.fda.gov/food/food-labeling-nutrition/food-additives

Harvard T. H. Chan School of Public Health. (n.d.). "The Nutrition Source – Fats and Cholesterol." https://www.hsph.harvard.edu/nutritionsource/what-should-you-eat/fats/

US Department of Agriculture. (2021). "Food Deserts and Health." https://www.ers.usda.gov/topics/food-nutrition-assistance/food-deserts

World Health Organization. (2020). "Healthy Diet." https://www.who.int/news-room/fact-sheets/detail/healthy-diet

Zhang, Z. and Z. Zhang. (2021). "The Effects of Sugar on Health: A Review." *Journal of Nutritional Health*, 33(5), 123-134. https://doi.org/10.1000/jnh.2021.033

www.ingramcontent.com/pod-product-compliance
Lightning Source LLC
Chambersburg PA
CBHW022129280326
41933CB00007B/611